LOW CARB DIET

HOW TO LOSE 7 POUNDS IN 7 DAYS WITH LOW CARB HIGH FAT DIET WITHOUT STARVING

SARAH E. DAWSON

Claim Your FREE Bonus!

As a token of appreciation for buying my book, I would like to give away a **FREE BONUS** report, *"10 Quick Weight Loss Tips and Tricks Revealed!"* just for you! May you gain more valuable insights in achieving your weight loss goals!

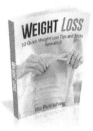

To claim your FREE bonus, simply go to the URL below:
http://bit.ly/weightloss-freebonus

Plus, by signing up to our subscription, you will also receive **FREE KINDLE BOOKS**, recipes, tips and tools to help you attain the weight you desire.

See you on the inside!

TABLE OF CONTENTS

INTRODUCTION

I want to thank you and congratulate you for buying the book, *"Low Carb Diet: How to Lose 7 Pounds in 7 Days with Low Carb High Fat Diet without Starving."*

The low carb diet is the go-to diet for those who want to shave off the excess weight without sacrificing taste and flavor. Aside from weight, conditions such as obesity, diabetes and cardiovascular diseases are becoming the most prevalent health concerns today. To minimize the risk and to combat the effects of these diseases, the low carb diet was created.

This book will give you information on the ideas behind the low carb diet, how it works and how you can benefit from it. There is also a useful section that will let you know which food items have the lowest carb count that you can use for your next recipe. It will also have a list of protein-rich food that you can also add into your meal plan. A dedicated section discusses the specific role of the low carb diet in relation to weight control with a "do-it-your-own" technique to measure and assess your weight. Additional information is also given for the different variations of diets that belong to the umbrella category of low carb diets.

The main section of the book is the 7 day meal plan. Each day of the plan has low carb recipes that are meant to be consumed for breakfast, lunch, dinner and a snack. In total, there are 28 recipes that you can choose from that are low carb diet friendly. The meal plan represents a wide range of food groups, meat, poultry, fish and vegan.

Begin your journey towards achieving your goal weight through the low carb diet!

Some of the topics in this book are:

- Overview of the diet

- Benefits and challenges

- Low carb food items

- High protein food items

- Various types of low carb diets

- 7 Day Meal Plan, each with Breakfast, Lunch, Dinner and a Snack

Thanks again for buying this book, I hope you enjoy it!

PART 1: THE LOW CARB DIET

Chapter 1: Introducing the Low Carb Diet

Overview of the Diet

Low carbohydrate or low carb diets are making their mark on the dietary world today. There is a wide variety of definitions for the low carb diet; some suggest that the limit is capped off at less than 20% of your intake of calories or a general reduction of your required carb consumption. Regardless of the definition, all low carb diets recommend that you reduce your carb intake, especially if you want to lose weight.

The secret behind the low carb diet is found on the relationship between carbohydrates, calories, and fats. When carbs are consumed, along with other food groups, they are converted into calories. These calories are meant to be the fuel of the body in performing its usual functions. The more active your lifestyle is, the more calories you burn. Calories that you do not use are stored as fat, which in turn is meant to be your reserve fuel for future use.

One of the best examples to illustrate this relationship is of the eating patterns of a bear. Prior to the winter season, a bear will consume vast amounts of food, more than he needs. This is because during the winter, it will be difficult for the bear to hunt. To keep his body nourished and functioning, the bear will store the food he consumed in the form of fat. When he hibernates, instead of eating, the body will use the stored fat.

The problem today is that the average person's lifestyle is slowly becoming more and more sedentary. This means when a person retains the same amount of carb intake but reduces their physical activity, more and more carbs are turned into calories that are unused. The more calories that are unused, the more fat is stored. This is where the low carb diet comes in to solve this problem. To cope with the decrease in caloric use, carb intake must also be limited.

Today, the low carb diet is being recommended by doctors, nutritionists, and other health professionals for patients with several kinds of diseases. Some of these diseases are high blood pressure, diabetes, and heart problems.

Benefits & Challenges

Aside from the health benefits, such as prevention and control of some diseases, the low carb diet is also known to have aesthetic contributions to those who adhere to its recommended meal plans. In fact, it is the weight loss benefit that attracts people more than its actual health benefits.

Weight control is made possible because it limits the formation of fat through the control of your carb intake. When you couple this diet with an active lifestyle, you can even burn unwanted fat. With the decrease of the formation of fat and the burning up of already stored fat in your body, the weight loss becomes even more possible and faster to achieve.

Aside from your body becoming leaner, your muscles also become stronger. The natural pair of low carb content is a high protein content diet. This means that not only are you able to remove excess fat, you can also tone your muscles into a better definition. The result is twofold, not only will your body look great but also your body will have more strength and endurance. The stronger you are, the more active your lifestyle can be, the more endurance you have, the longer you can perform your exercises. This combination creates the perfect situation, a diet that makes your body not only look good but also feel good and function well.

Another benefit is that as the name implies, it does not totally restrict you from eating carbs. Instead, it only minimizes your carb intake. This means that you can still enjoy your favorite carb foods. Taste, flavor, and a feeling of fullness can still be achieved in this diet. This is also another reason why most people prefer the low carb diet over others. Some diets totally restrict certain food groups, which in turn sacrifices taste and satisfaction. With the low carb diet, you do not have to starve. In fact, the food tastes better aside from actually being healthy alternatives themselves.

There are however some challenges in the low carb diet. First is the adjustment phase. You may find yourself getting tired easily in the first few weeks of the diet. This is because of your decreased source of calories. This effect is temporary and when your body has adjusted to the diet, you will actually feel more energized because your digestive system is now processing the amount it is meant to digest. Your absorption becomes better and metabolism reaches ideal levels.

Another challenge is that some of the diet's recommended ingredients are more expensive. For example, instead of any fish, the low carb diet recommends salmon. Instead of any part of meat or poultry, you are required to choose the leaner or choice cut versions. On the other hand, you can still opt to have the cheaper but still equally low carb content choices. For example, instead of salmon you can buy tilapia, a kind of white fish that is also called "the poor man's fish."

Take note, as with any other diet, the low carb diet is not meant to be a substitute for any physical exercise or medication that you are taking. Diets are meant to augment and not to replace your health choices. Diets work best when they are practiced in conjunction with other healthy choices. For example, you can quickly reach your desired weight if you pair the low carb diet with a routine exercise. If you plan to follow this diet, it is best to consult your doctor, especially if you have medical conditions.

Chapter 2: Low-Carb Friendly Food Groups & Weight Loss

Low Carb Food Groups

Take this list with you on your next trip to the grocery and make the right choices. The food items listed below have some of the lowest carb content. Make these items the main ingredients of your recipes.

These food items are:

For vegetables
- Zucchini
- Cauliflower
- Mushrooms
- Celery
- Cherry tomatoes
- Squash

For fruits
- Avocado
- Strawberries
- Peaches
- Cantaloupe

- Watermelon

For fish

- Catfish
- Halibut
- Tilapia
- Salmon

For poultry

- Chicken thighs
- Ground turkey
- Chicken breast

For meat

- Sirloin steak
- Pork tenderloin
- Roast beef

For other food items

- Eggs
- Cottage cheese
- Greek yogurt, plain
- Walnuts
- Jerky
- Almond flour

High Protein Food Groups

Below are some food items that have high protein contents:

- Cottage cheese
- Greek yogurt
- Eggs
- Milk
- Steak
- Ground beef
- Chicken breast
- Turkey breast
- Tilapia
- Tuna
- Salmon
- Halibut
- Anchovies
- Sardines
- Chorizo
- Bacon
- Peanuts
- Almonds
- Watermelon seeds
- Pumpkin seeds

- Beans
- Quinoa
- Tofu
- Soy milk

Weight Control & BMI

If weight control is your objective for the low carb diet, then you must know your ideal body weight and the interpretation of your current body weight. One of most widely used tools to measure your ideal weight is through the Body Mass Index or BMI formula.

To calculate BMI:

1. Weigh yourself using pounds as your measurement
2. Measure your height using inches
3. Multiply the number of inches with itself
4. Divide the result with your weight
5. Multiply the result with 703

For example, if you measure 60 inches and 100 pounds then:

1. 60 x 60 = 3600
2. 100 / 3600 = .03
3. .03 x 703 = 21.09

Refer to the table below to determine your BMI:

18.6 and below = underweight

18.7 to 24.8= ideal weight

24.9 to 29.9 = overweight

30 and above = obesity

If the result of your BMI is either underweight or obesity, consider consulting your doctor before starting the low carb diet plan. If you follow the diet and you are underweight, you may push your body to its limits. Too much fat is just as bad as too little because fat is meant to be used as emergency food of the body, especially during sleep. If you follow the diet and you are obese, you need to control the amount of weight that you lose. This is because your body may not be able to cope with the sudden drop in weight. When in doubt, it is better to seek professional help, especially if you belong to one of the extremes of the BMI scale.

Each person is unique with their own health background and situation; this means that with the low carb diet, the weight loss will also be different. For some, especially those with an active lifestyle, the weight loss will be more significant compared to those who only rely on the diet for the reduction of their weight.

This means that in this diet plan, you may not lose as much as 7 pounds. But one thing is for sure, under this diet, you will sure to lose unwanted weight. Use every weight loss as motivation towards sustaining the diet. You may not reach your ideal weight within a week's time but given time and discipline, you will have the weight that you truly deserve.

Chapter 3: Low Carb Diet Types

The low carb diet is actually an umbrella term for the various types of diets that encourage reduction of carb consumption with a goal to have a healthier lifestyle and to reduce weight. While there are a variety of low carb diets, each with their own principles, rules, and recommendations, they all share the low-carb basis.

Some of the more popular low carb variants are:

1. Atkins
2. Stillman
3. Hollywood
4. Zone
5. Dukan

Atkins Diet

Arguably the most popular low carb diet, the Atkins diet is the product of Dr. Robert Atkins. With an overweight condition himself, Atkins wanted to address and solve his weight problem. His weight loss method has been widely practiced and has provided various results.

The Atkins diet shares the same principles with the low carb diet because it significantly reduces the daily intake of carbs in meals. The low carb principles are translated into the four phases of the Atkins diet: induction, ongoing weight loss, pre-maintenance, and lifetime maintenance.

Induction is potentially the most difficult phase of the diet because it totally restricts followers from consuming any carb, or caps the intake to less than 20 grams a day. Within 2 weeks of this phase, the body consumes your fat content thereby reducing your weight. The next phase is the ongoing weight loss where the follower consumes incremental amounts of carbs until they reach their desired weight.

Once the weight is achieved, pre-maintenance phase follows, where the exact amount of carbs that do not allow weight gain is consumed. Once this quantity of carb is established, followers can start with the lifetime maintenance. This represents applying all the lessons learned from the previous phases, eating just enough carbs but still without gaining weight.

Stillman Diet

Named after its creator, Dr. Irwin Stillman, this diet is also low carb but not as restrictive as the Atkins diet. This diet actually came before the famous Atkins diet. Stillman was a doctor that specialized in obesity and he was regularly consulted by overweight patients.

Although it does not allow butter, dressings, fats or oils, this diet has no restrictions on consumption of lean beef, fish, poultry, eggs, spices, tea, and coffee. Preparation is also monitored; recipes are mostly baked, boiled, or broiled. Emphasis is also given on drinking 8 full glasses of water and 7 small meals per day instead of a 3 large meals.

One criticism of the diet is that it does not allow enough fiber content in its recipes, resulting in an unbalanced diet. While it does offer weight reduction to more than 15 lbs in the first week of the diet alone, most followers need supplements of the nutrients they do not get from the limited food items.

Hollywood Diet

Named the Hollywood diet because it was created by Jamie Kabler, a popular nutritionist for Hollywood celebrities, this diet gained its reputation because of its promise of success within a short period of time. Instead of consuming low carb solid foods, this diet offers an orange-colored drink. This drink is a combination of various fruits' juice concentrates and is the only food source for at least 2 days.

After the consumption of this drink, the follower can undergo the Hollywood diet's 30-day miracle program. This program is meant to provide followers with the same weight loss benefits of the 2-day drink but this time with solid foods and with a meal that uses a Hollywood diet program product, such as the Mix Meal, the Meta Miracle, and other products.

Zone Diet

Aside from focusing on carbs alone, the Zone diet takes into consideration the role of insulin in weight. According to this diet, insulin, a hormone that balances blood sugar levels, is guilty for storing fat, which in turn increases weight. To control weight, the theory is you need to control your insulin levels. When dieters keep their insulin levels at the bare minimum, fat is burned and therefore more weight is lost.

This is where carbs come into the diet. When carbs are controlled, or also kept at a minimum but with an adequate consumption of protein and fats, insulin is controlled. This perfect balance of protein, fats, carbs, and insulin is referred to as the zone. This diet shows that followers can lose at least 5 pounds per week.

Dukan Diet

Although the Dukan diet has the same phases as with the Atkins diet, it is stricter. While the first phase of the Atkins allows a very minimal carb consumption, in the Dukan, even vegetables that are already low-carb are not allowed. Further restrictions include eggs, steaks, and pork chops. The focus on this diet shifts to the importance of protein together with the elimination of carbs.

The idea behind the diet is that to maximize weight loss potential, aside from eliminating carbs, increased protein intake will reduce more weight. This is because the body requires more energy to break down and digest protein. At the same time, protein takes longer to digest and this allows the feeling of a full stomach to last longer. The result is that you burn more fats to digest proteins and you can also delay feelings of hunger longer than usual.

PART 2: THE 7 DAY MEAL PLAN

Chapter 4: Ready, get set, lose! A burst of flavors to start your weight loss week

Day One Meal Plan

Breakfast: Egg & Spinach

Lunch: Coconut Beef

Dinner: Chicken Skewers

Snacks: Choco Mousse

Eggs & Spinach

Servings: 4

Ingredients:

- 4 eggs
- 10 oz. spinach
- 3 tbsp leek, chopped
- 1 tsp lemon juice
- 2 tbsp scallion, chopped
- 2 tbsp butter, divided
- 1 clove garlic, halved
- 1 tsp oregano, chopped
- 1/4 tsp red pepper flakes
- 1/4 tsp paprika

- 2/3 cup plain Greek yogurt
- 2 tbsp olive oil
- Salt and pepper

Directions:

1. Heat oven to 300 degrees
2. Put skillet on medium heat and add butter
3. Add scallion and leek then set heat to low
4. Cook for 10 minutes
5. Add lemon juice and spinach
6. Add salt to taste
7. Cook for another 5 minutes on high and turn the spinach until they wilt
8. Transfer mixture to another skillet and make sure to leave liquid
9. Use a spoon to make indentations on the mixture and crack the eggs into each indentation
10. Bake for 15 minutes
11. Put saucepan on low heat and melt remaining butter
12. Sprinkle pepper flakes, paprika and salt and cook for another 2 minutes
13. Add oregano
14. Combine garlic, salt and yogurt in a bowl and set aside
15. Take garlic mixture and scoop garlic leaving only the yoghurt mixture

16. Spread mixture on top of baked eggs and drizzle with melted butter
17. Serve

Coconut Beef

Servings: 4

Ingredients:

- 1 lb. steak, cut into thin strips
- 1 lb. pack of mixed stir fry vegetables
- 9 oz. rice noodles
- 3 tbsp red curry paste
- 4 tbsp coriander, chopped
- 2 tsp groundnut oil
- 9 oz. coconut milk
- 2 tbsp lime juice
- 1 tsp sugar

Directions:

1. Put together sugar, lime juice and paste with steak. Marinate for 5 minutes.
2. Place pan over medium heat and add marinated steak. Fry for 2 minutes.
3. Add milk and bring to a boil
4. Add vegetables and cook for another 5 minutes
5. Cook the noodles
6. Put noodles on bowl, top with the beef mixture
7. Top with coriander
8. Serve

Chicken Skewers

Servings: 3

Ingredients:

- ½ lb. chicken breast, cut into fillets
- 1 green pepper, remove the seeds
- 1 tbsp lemon juice
- 6 tbsp plain yogurt
- 2 tbsp curry paste
- 1 ripe mango, diced
- 1 tbsp lime juice
- 2 onions, chopped
- Salt and pepper

Directions:

1. Heat grill to medium for 15 minutes
2. Put together paste, lemon juice, yogurt and salt on shallow plate, mix well and set side
3. Cut the fillets into chunks and add into the yogurt mixture. Toss until the fillets are well coated.
4. Marinate the chicken for an hour while covered
5. Cut the pepper into squares. Skewer chicken and pepper in alternating order.
6. Put on grill and turn skewers to cook on all sides
7. Remove from grill when chicken is charred
8. Put together lime juice, onions and mango together, add salt and pepper to taste

9. Serve with mango salsa on the side

Choco Mousse

Servings: 4

Ingredients:

- 1 1/2 cups heavy cream
- 6 packets Equal sugar substitute
- 1/2 teaspoon vanilla extract
- 1/4 cup unsweetened cocoa powder

Directions:

1. Whip the cream with electric mixer.

2. Add Equal one packet at a time.

3. Add vanilla and cocoa powder, and beat until almost stiff.

4. Scrape down and mix again.

5. Place in serving dishes, cover, and refrigerate for at least 1/2 hour.

6. Serve within 4 hours of preparation.

Chapter 5: Here it comes! First pound down! Power meals without the guilt

Day Two Meal Plan

Breakfast: Pancakes

Lunch: Roast Chicken

Dinner: Salmon Frittatas

Snacks: Power Drink

Pancakes

Servings: 2

Ingredients:

- 1/2 cup besan flour
- 1 onion, chopped
- 1 tbsp olive oil
- 1/4 tsp garlic powder
- 1/4 tsp baking powder
- 1/2 cup water
- Salt and pepper

Direction:

1. Combine besan flour, baking powder, garlic powder, and salt and pepper in a bowl. Whisk together until completely mixed.

2. Add water and mix again, make sure there are no clumps

3. Put the vegetables in the mixture, set aside

4. Heat skillet to medium and add olive oil

5. Put the mixture and spread on the skillet. Cook each side for 5 minutes.

6. If desired, top with avocado, cashew, or other fruits and nuts

7. Serve

Roast Chicken

Servings: 4

Ingredients:

- 4 chicken breasts, skinned and deboned
- 1 onion, sliced
- 2 cloves garlic, diced
- 2 tbsp olive oil
- 1 cup tomatoes, diced
- 1 cup black olives, pitted and drained
- ½ tsp cumin
- ½ tsp paprika
- ½ tsp salt
- ½ tsp pepper

Directions:

1. Heat oven to 350 degrees
2. Place pan over high heat and add olive oil
3. Add garlic and onion to pan and sauté for 2 minutes
4. Add olives, tomatoes, and chicken
5. Put together cumin, paprika, and salt and pepper in a small bowl and then sprinkle on top of chicken while cooking
6. Put pan inside oven and bake for 30 minutes
7. Serve

Salmon Frittatas

Servings: 3

Ingredients:

- 2 oz. salmon, cut into ¼ inch pieces
- 3 eggs
- 4 egg whites
- 1 tbsp scallions, sliced into thin pieces
- 1/8 cup onion, diced
- ½ tbsp half and half
- 2 tbsp milk
- 2 oz. fat free cream cheese, cubed
- Salt and pepper

Directions:

1. Heat oven to 325 degrees
2. Place skillet on high heat and add oil
3. Sauté onions for 2 minutes
4. Add salmon and salt and pepper and then remove from heat
5. Put eggs, egg whites, half and half and milk in a bowl
6. Stir together with cheese
7. Spray ramekins with cooking spray
8. Scoop 2 tbsp of salmon mixture into ramekin
9. Pour egg mixture on top of salmon and fill until below the rim
10. Bake ramekins for 25 minutes and serve.

Power Drink

Servings: 2

Ingredients:

- 1 avocado
- ½ cup Greek yogurt
- 1 tsp green tea powder
- ¼ cup protein powder, vanilla flavor
- ¼ cup almond milk, unsweetened
- 2 tsp sweetener
- 1 tbsp hot water

Directions:

1. Mix together tea powder and hot water, set aside
2. Cut the avocado into chunks and put in blender
3. Add sweetener, yogurt, and protein powder into blender
4. Pour milk and tea mixture into blender
5. Blend into smooth consistency
6. Serve

Chapter 6: Keep it going, total lost- 2 to 3 pounds, reward yourself with these low-carb comfort food

Day Three Meal Plan

Breakfast: Quinoa Bowl

Lunch: Beef Stew

Dinner: Buffalo Chicken

Snacks: Crepes

Quinoa Bowl

Servings: 4

Ingredients:

- 4 eggs
- 1 cup quinoa
- 1 avocado, chopped
- 6 oz. salmon, smoked
- 2 tbsp olive oil
- 1 cup scallion, sliced
- 1 tbsp lemon juice
- Salt and pepper

Directions:

1. Cook quinoa, while it is cooking, heat skillet on medium
2. Cook eggs for 5 minutes, add salt and pepper to taste
3. Take the quinoa and layer with eggs first, then avocado, and then salmon cuts
4. Drizzle with the juice
5. Garnish with scallions
6. Serve

Beef Stew

Servings: 4

Ingredients:

- 2 lbs. beef chuck roast, cut into cubes
- 8 oz tomato sauce
- 14.5 oz tomatoes with juice, diced
- 1 can low sodium beef broth
- 1 tbsp olive oil
- 1 cup cloves garlic, cut into slivers
- 2 tbsp capers
- 3 tbsp red wine vinegar
- 3 bay leaves
- 1 tsp oregano
- 1 cup olives cut into half
- Salt and pepper

Directions:

1. Add 1 tbsp of oil to pan over high heat
2. Cook beef cubes until they are brown on all sides
3. Put cubes in slow cooker and set aside
4. Pour broth into pan where cubes were cooked and simmer
5. Pour broth into slow cooker
6. Add remaining ingredients: olives, garlic, capers, oregano, tomatoes, vinegar, pepper, bay leaves and sauce into slow cooker

7. Set to high and cook for 4 hours
8. Serve

Buffalo Chicken

Servings: 2

Ingredients:

- 5 chicken thighs, skinned
- 1 tsp seasoning
- 1/3 cup blue cheese
- 1 tbsp olive oil
- 1 tbsp Worcestershire sauce
- 1 tsp mustard
- 1 tsp hot sauce
- ½ tsp garlic powder
- ½ tsp onion powder
- 1 tbsp brown sugar
- Salt and pepper

Directions:

1. Heat oven to 400 degrees
2. Spray oil in baking dish
3. Trim the chicken of any fat and put in baking dish
4. Sprinkle seasoning, salt and pepper
5. Bake chicken for 15 minutes
6. Combine olive oil, Worcestershire sauce, mustard, sugar and onion and garlic powder together
7. Turn the chicken every 15 minutes, once turned glaze the sauce on each side. Repeat 3 times.

8. On the fourth time it is glazed, add the cheese on top and let it cook for another 10 minutes

9. Serve

Crepes

Servings: 3

Ingredients:
- 2 eggs
- 2 egg whites
- ½ tsp baking soda
- ¼ cup coconut flour
- ¼ cup almond milk, unsweetened
- 2 tbsp flaxseed
- Choice of berries

Directions:
1. Heat skillet on high and coat with cooking spray
2. Mix all ingredients in a blender
3. Blend until completely combined
4. Pour mixture into skillet and completely cover it with the batter
5. Allow to cook until bubbles form and pop on top
6. After 3 minutes, flip crepe and cook the other side
7. Put berries inside the crepe and a few whole pieces on top
8. Serve

Chapter 7: Halfway there, total pounds lost- 3 to 4! Classic meals with a low carb twist

Day Four Meal Plan

Breakfast: Muffins

Lunch: Meatballs

Dinner: Tuna Patties

Snacks: Berry Parfaits

Muffins

Servings: 12

Ingredients:

- 6 eggs
- 1 onion, thinly sliced
- ½ cup low fat cottage cheese
- ½ cup almond flour
- ½ cup parmesan cheese, grated
- ¼ cup flax seed
- ¼ cup yeast flakes
- ½ cup hemp seed
- Salt

Directions:

1. Heat oven to 375 degrees
2. Spray muffin pans with oil
3. In a large bowl, mix almond, cheese, flax seed, yeast flakes, baking powder, hemp seed, and salt and set aside
4. In a separate bowl, mix eggs, cheese, and onions
5. Mix together powder mixture with egg mixture
6. Put combined mixture into muffin cups
7. Bake for 30 minutes
8. Serve

Meatballs

Servings: 36 meatballs

Ingredients:

- 1 lb lean ground beef
- 1 lb lean ground turkey
- ½ tsp allspice
- ½ tsp cardamom
- ¼ tsp cinnamon
- ¼ tsp white pepper
- ½ tsp ginger
- 1 tbsp garlic
- 1 onion
- Salt

Directions:

1. Heat oven to 400 degrees
2. Put both ground beef and turkey in a bowl and set aside
3. Chop onion and put in with meats, cinnamon, cardamom, garlic, ginger, salt and pepper, combine thoroughly
4. Spray oil on grilling rack
5. Form balls by rolling mixture into your hands and place them on grill
6. Bake for 30 minutes

7. Serve

Tuna Patties

Servings: 1

Ingredients:

- 1 can of tuna, light
- 1 egg
- ¼ tsp garlic powder
- 1 tbsp onion, chopped
- ¼ tsp salt

Directions:

1. Put pan on medium heat and spray with oil

2. Place all ingredients in a bowl and mix together

3. Divide mixture into 6 and scoop each into pan

4. Flatten in a size just enough to flip with a spatula

5. Cook both sides

6. Serve

Berry Parfaits

Servings: 3

Ingredients:

- 8 oz milk ricotta
- 1 tsp lemon zest
- 2 tbsp lemon juice
- 8 drops extract of stevia
- 1 cup of berries of choice

Directions:

1. Put stevia, zest, juice, and ricotta in blender, mix for 2 minutes
2. Use clear glasses and make alternate layers of berries and ricotta mixture
3. Serve

Chapter 8: The goal is in sight! Full speed ahead with these easy recipes

Day Five Meal Plan

Breakfast: Breakfast Bake

Lunch: White fish and capers

Dinner: Chicken Pesto

Snacks: Cookies

Breakfast Bake

Servings: 4

Ingredients:

- 12 turkey sausages
- ½ cup low fat mozzarella, grated
- 1 red bell pepper, chopped
- 1 green bell pepper, chopped
- 2 tsp olive oil
- Pepper

Directions:
1. Heat oven to 450 degrees
2. Cut red and green bell peppers into 1 inch slices

3. Spray baking dish with oil and put peppers on the dish

4. Bake for 20 minutes

5. Put pan on high heat and add oil

6. Cook sausages for 10 minutes

7. Cut sausages into 1/3 size and add with the peppers in the oven

8. Bake for another 5 minutes

9. Take sausages from the oven and sprinkle cheese

10. Put in oven and set to broil

11. Broil for 2 minutes

12. Serve

White Fish and Capers

Servings: 3

Ingredients:

- 3 tilapia fillets
- ¼ cup parmesan cheese, grated
- 2 tbsp olive oil
- 1 lemon
- 2 tbsp capers and brine
- Salt and pepper

Directions:

1. Place fillets on a plate and drizzle 1 tbsp oil on all fillets, both sides
2. Sprinkle salt and pepper on fillets, set aside
3. Put cheese in a wide bowl, set aside
4. Put pan on medium heat and add 1 tbsp of oil
5. Dredge fillets through cheese and then put in pan
6. Cook each fillet for 5 minutes on each side
7. Add capers in pan when time is almost up
8. Squeeze lemon on fish
9. Serve

Chicken pesto

Servings: 3

Ingredients:

- 2 chicken breasts, skinned and deboned
- 1 onion
- 1 can chicken broth
- ½ can water
- 2 zucchini
- 1/3 cup pesto
- 2 tsp. all-purpose seasoning
- 1/3 cup vinaigrette dressing
- Salt and pepper

Directions:

1. Simmer broth and water in a saucepan
2. Add chicken and cook for 20 minutes
3. Remove chicken from broth and set aside
4. Mix together pesto, dressing, seasoning, and pepper, set aside
5. Cut chicken and into cubes
6. Put chicken cubes and ¼ cup of pesto mixture together in a container
7. Marinate for 1 hour
8. Slice onions and zucchini into thin slices and put into bowl
9. Add remaining pesto sauce with the vegetables

10. Plate the chicken and serve

Cookies

Servings: 20

Ingredients:

- 1 egg
- 1 cup peanut butter
- 1 cup sweetener

Directions:

1. Heat oven to 350 degrees

2. Put all ingredients in a bowl and mix together

3. Roll mixture into 20 separate balls

4. Bake for 10 minutes

5. Serve

Chapter 9: Hang in there, easy recipes to get you going for the final push!

Day Six Meal Plan

Breakfast: Oatmeal

Lunch: Chinese Chicken

Dinner: Mushroom Polenta

Snacks: Ceviche

Oatmeal

Servings: 4

Ingredients:

- 2 tbsp cinnamon
- ½ cup unsweetened coconut, shredded into fine pieces
- ½ cup golden flax
- ½ cup chia seeds
- 2 tbsp unsweetened coconut milk
- ½ cup water
- Sweetener
- Berries of choice

Directions:

1. Mix flax, coconut, chia, and cinnamon

2. Scoop ½ cup of the mixture and add water, set aside for 5 minutes
3. Add milk and desired amount of sweetener and stir
4. Top with berries and serve

Chinese Chicken

Servings: 4

Ingredients:

Chicken ingredients

- 1 lb. chicken thighs, deboned and skinned
- 1/4 tsp garlic powder
- 1/4 tsp onion powder
- 1/8 cup soy sauce
- 1 tsp ginger
- 2 cups water

Salad ingredients

- 1 cup cucumbers, sliced
- 1 cup Napa cabbage, shredded
- 1 cup white cabbage, shredded
- 1/4 cup scallions, sliced
- 1/8 cup cilantro, chopped
- 1 tbsp sesame seeds
- 1/4 cup radishes cut into thin slices
- Dressing ingredients
- 1/8 cup soy sauce
- 1/8 tsp Chinese mustard
- 1/2 tsp sesame oil
- 1/8 cup rice wine vinegar
- 1/2 tbsp sweetener
- 2 tbsp avocado oil
- 1/2 tbsp ginger paste

Directions:

1. Put chicken, garlic, onion powder, soy sauce, ginger, and water in saucepan. Bring to a boil.

2. Lower heat and simmer for 20 minutes

3. Remove chicken and shred, remove any remaining fat or ligaments, set aside

4. Put the cabbages in a bowl and keep the center portion empty for the chicken

5. Add the cilantro, radishes, and scallions

6. Add the chicken in the middle

7. Sprinkle seeds on top and serve

Mushroom Polenta

Servings: 4

Ingredients:

- 8 flat mushrooms
- 2 cups goat cheese
- 500 g pack of polenta, sliced
- 50 g bag of rocket leaves
- 4 tbsp olive oil
- 75 g peppers, chopped
- 2 tbsp oregano
- Salt and pepper

Directions:

1. Put mushrooms in a bowl and drizzle oil on top

2. Heat grill to medium and cook mushrooms for 5 minutes, remove from heat

3. Sprinkle the oregano and add the peppers

4. Add the cheese

5. Put back on grill and wait for cheese to melt

6. Add the polenta on the grill and cook for 5 minutes each side

7. Top the polenta with rocket leaves

8. Add salt and pepper to taste

9. Serve

Ceviche

Servings: 3

Ingredients:

- 8 oz. button mushrooms, sliced into thin pieces
- ½ vegetable broth
- 1/3 cup lemon juice
- ½ red bell pepper, sliced into thin strips
- ½ green bell pepper, sliced into thin strips
- 1 onion, sliced
- 2 cloves garlic
- 1 tbsp cilantro, chopped
- ¼ tsp honey
- 1 tsp jalapeno, chopped
- 1 tbsp olive oil
- Salt and pepper

Directions:

1. Sauté garlic in a skillet over medium heat for 2 minutes
2. Mash garlic and then put in bowl, add onion, red and green peppers and mushrooms, set aside
3. Put together all ingredients in a separate bowl, mix well
4. Pour seasoning into mushroom mixture
5. Put in covered container and refrigerate overnight
6. Serve

Chapter 10: Wait for it, wait for it- 6 to 7 pounds down! Congratulations!

Day Seven Meal Plan

Breakfast: Veggie Hash

Lunch: Meatloaf

Dinner: Shrimp Salad

Snacks: Pepper Poppers

Veggie Hash

Servings: 2

Ingredients:

- ¾ lb cauliflower, cut into small pieces
- 1 onion
- 2 tbsp olive oil
- 1 clove garlic, minced
- 2 tsp lemon juice
- ¼ tsp paprika
- 3 tbsp water
- Salt and pepper

Directions:

1. Add oil to skillet over high heat

2. Cook onion and cauliflower without stirring for 3 minutes

3. Add paprika, salt, pepper, and water

4. Cover skillet and cook for another 5 minutes

5. Reduce heat to low and add garlic, cook for another 2 minutes while stirring

6. Add lemon juice and cook for another 30 seconds

7. Serve

Meatloaf

Servings: 4

Ingredients:

- 1 lb ground beef lean
- 3 eggs
- 1/2 cup shredded cheese
- 4 oz green pepper, diced
- 1/8 cup sour cream
- 1 clove garlic
- 1/4 tsp cumin
- 1/2 tsp chili powder

Directions:

1. Heat oven to 400 degrees

2. Whisk eggs in bowl and set aside

3. Put beef in bowl, add eggs, cumin, and chili powder

4. Use a waxed paper and roll the beef mixture halfway, create a flat square

5. Put half of the chili and cheese on top

6. Roll the other side until it becomes a loaf

7. Remove the wax paper

8. Fold ends of the loaf to keep the chili and cheese from spilling

9. Put loaf in pan and top with the remaining chili, cheese, and the cream

10. Bake for 1 hour

11. Serve

Salmon & Shrimp Salad

Servings: 1

Ingredients:

- 100 g salmon, cut into bite size pieces, cooked
- 1 cup spinach
- 1 cup watercress
- 10 prawns, cooked
- 100 g Greek yogurt
- 2 tsp dill
- 1 tsp lemon juice
- 1 lemon wedge

Directions:

1. Put yogurt, zest from lemon wedge, dill, and pepper together in a bowl, mix together and set aside
2. Put together vegetables with the salmon
3. Add prawns and scoop yogurt dressing on top
4. Serve

Pepper Poppers

Servings: 4

Ingredients:

- ½ lb baby peppers
- 4 oz bacon, chopped and cooked
- 1 tbsp hot sauce
- 1 tbsp cilantro, chopped
- 2 avocados
- 1 tbsp lime juice
- Salt

Directions:

1. Heat oven to 350 degrees
2. Remove the stem of the peppers and cut the peppers lengthwise
3. Remove seeds and membrane
4. Put peppers on baking sheet and cook for 10 minutes
5. Mash avocados and combine with hot sauce, cilantro, and juice
6. Add salt to taste
7. Scoop guacamole and fill hollow part of the pepper
8. Sprinkle with bacon and serve

Chapter 11: More LCHF Recipes

Breakfast Recipes

Hashbrown Potato Cakes

Serves 8

Ingredients:

- 1 pound russet or round red potatoes
- 1/2 of a medium onion, very thinly sliced
- 1 tablespoon olive oil
- 2 teaspoons snipped fresh thyme or 1/4 teaspoon dried thyme, crushed
- 1/4 teaspoon salt
- 1/8 teaspoon ground black pepper
- Nonstick cooking spray

Directions:
1. Preheat oven to 300 degrees F.
2. Peel and coarsely shred potatoes; immediately rinse with cold water in a colander.

3. Drain well, pressing lightly, then pat dry with paper towels; place in a large bowl. Quarter the onion slices. Stir onion, oil, thyme, salt, and pepper into potatoes.

4. Lightly coat an unheated very large nonstick skillet or griddle with nonstick cooking spray.

5. Preheat skillet or griddle over medium heat.

6. For each cake, scoop a slightly rounded measuring tablespoon of the potato mixture onto skillet or griddle.

7. Press down potato mixture with a spatula to flatten evenly. Cook for 5 minutes. Using a wide spatula, carefully turn potato cakes (be sure not to turn cakes too soon or they will not hold together).

8. Cook for 3 to 5 minutes more or until golden brown.

9. Place cooked potato cakes on a baking sheet.

10. Keep warm, uncovered, in oven while cooking remaining potato cakes.

11. Repeat with remaining potato mixture, stirring mixture frequently.

Low Carb Pizza Waffles

Serves 5

Ingredients:

- 5 eggs separated
- 4 tbs coconut flour
- salt to taste
- 1 tbs dried herbs of choice - I use rosemary and oregano
- 1 tsp baking powder
- 125g / 4.5oz/ 1 stick + 1 tbs butter, melted
- 3 tbs full fat milk
- ½ cup grated cheese

Directions:

1. Whisk the egg whites until firm and form stiff peaks.
2. In a separate bowl, mix the egg yolks, coconut flour, salt, herbs and baking powder.
3. Add the melted butter slowly, mixing to ensure it is a smooth consistency.
4. Add the milk and grated cheese. Mix well.

5. Gently fold spoons of the whisked egg whites into the yolk mixture. Try to keep as much of the air and volume as possible.

6. Place enough of the waffle mixture into the warm waffle maker to make one waffle. Cook until golden.

7. Repeat until all the mixture has been used

Low Carb Egg Salad

Serves 4

Ingredients:

- 6 hard boiled eggs
- ½ cup full fat mayonnaise
- ½ - 1 tsp curry powder to taste

Directions:
1. To make the boiled eggs, place the eggs in a saucepan and cover with COLD water.
2. Turn the heat on and once the water begins to boil, let them boil for 7 minutes.
3. Drain and cover with cold water to stop them from cooking further.
4. Once cool, peel and chop the eggs into small pieces.
5. Mix the eggs, mayonnaise and curry powder.
6. Serve with chopped fresh parsley.

Breakfast Tacos

Serving 2 tacos

Ingredients:

- 22 eggs
- 1/8 tsp.1 g oregano
- 1/8 tsp.1 g cumin
- Salt and pepper
- 22 low carb tortillas
- 2 tbsp.18.75 g avocado
- 2 tbsp.1 g salsa

Directions:

1. Spray a microwave safe dish with cooking spray.
2. Whisk together the eggs, cumin, oregano salt, and pepper. If you are adding extra veggies stir them in as well. If your veggies are raw, you can microwave them first for 1-2 minutes until just tender.
3. Microwave the eggs for 1 minute. Remove and scramble with your fork. Return to microwave for 1-1.5 minutes until cooked through.
4. Microwave the tortillas for 10-15 seconds.
5. Assemble your tacos with your favorite salsa, avocado, and any additional toppings.

Cinnamon Roll Scones

Serves 8

Ingredients:

Scones:

- 2 cups almond flour
- 3 tbsp Swerve Sweetener
- 2 tsp baking powder
- 1/2 tsp salt
- 1/4 tsp ground cinnamon
- 1 large egg, lightly beaten
- 1/4 cup coconut oil, melted (butter may be substituted)
- 2 tbsp heavy cream
- 1/2 tsp vanilla extract

Filling/Topping:

- 3 tbsp Swerve Sweetener
- 2 tsp cinnamon

Icing:

- 1 oz cream cheese, softened
- 1 tbsp cream

- 1/2 tbsp butter, softened
- 1 tbsp powdered Swerve Sweetener
- 1/4 tsp vanilla extract

Directions:

Scones:

1. Line a baking sheet with parchment paper and preheat oven to 325F. Whisk together almond flour, sweetener, baking powder, salt and cinnamon in a large bowl. Add in egg, coconut oil, cream, and vanilla extract until dough comes together.

2. In a small bowl, whisk together filling ingredients. Sprinkle half of filling into dough and mix in, but do not fully incorporate, so that it remains streaky.

3. Turn out dough onto parchment-lined baking sheet and shape by hand into a rough circle, 7 or 8 inches in diameter. Sprinkle with remaining topping. Slice into 8 even wedges and separate carefully, then space evenly around the baking sheet. Bake 20 to 25 minutes, or until scones are firm and lightly browned. Keep an eye on the bottoms to make sure they don't burn.

4. Remove from oven, transfer to a wire rack and let it cool.

Icing:

1. Beat cream cheese, butter and cream together until smooth.
2. Beat in powdered sweetener and vanilla extract until combined.
3. Pipe or spread over cooled scones.

Lemon Ricotta Pancakes

Ingredients:

Mixed Berry Syrup:

- 1 cup mixed frozen berries (raspberries, blueberries, blackberries, strawberries)
- 1/4 cup water
- Sugar equivalent to 2 tbsp sugar
- 1/4 tsp xanthan gum

Pancakes:

- 3/4 cup ricotta
- 3 large eggs
- 1/4 cup lemon juice
- 1/4 cup water
- Zest of one lemon
- 1 1/2 cups almond flour
- Sweetener equivalent to 1/4 cup sugar
- 2 tbsp coconut flour
- 1 1/2 tsp baking powder
- 1/4 tsp salt
- Butter or oil for the pan

Directions:

Syrup:

1. In a medium saucepan over medium heat, combine berries, water and sweetener.

2. Bring to a boil, then reduce heat and simmer until berries are soft enough to be mashed with a fork.

3. Sprinkle with xanthan gum and whisk vigorously to combine. Set aside to thicken.

Pancakes:

1. In a blender, combine ricotta, eggs, lemon juice, water and lemon zest. Blend until well mixed, about 10 seconds.

2. Add almond flour, sweetener, coconut flour, baking powder and salt and blend until mixture is smooth (if using a coarser almond meal, you will need to blend it for 30 seconds to a minute).

3. Heat a griddle or large skillet over medium heat and add butter or oil. Once pan is hot, spoon about 3 tbsp of batter into 4 inch circles and let cook until edges look dry, a few small bubbles appear on the top, and the underside is golden brown. Flip carefully and continue to cook until second side is golden brown, about 2 to 3 minutes.

4. Remove and keep pancakes warm while repeating with remaining batter. You should get about 12 pancakes.

5. Serve pancakes with butter and mixed berry syrup.

Lunch Recipes

Broccoli Slaw Pasta

Serves 2

Ingredients:

- 1 12-ounce bag (4 cups) dry broccoli slaw
- 1 cup low-fat creamy tomato soup (like Amy's Chunky Tomato Bisque) or canned crushed tomatoes
- 1 teaspoon chopped garlic or more, to taste
- Dash onion powder or more, to taste
- Dash each salt and black pepper or more, to taste
- Dash crushed red pepper or more, to taste
- 3 tablespoons reduced-fat parmesan-style grated topping, divided

Directions:

1. Bring a skillet sprayed with nonstick spray to medium-high heat on the stove.
2. Add slaw and 1/4 cup water. Stirring occasionally, cook until water has evaporated and slaw has softened slightly, about 5 to 8 minutes.

3. Add soup/tomatoes, garlic, spices, and 2 tablespoons grated topping. Stir, and continue to cook until hot, about 3 to 4 minutes.

4. Season to taste with additional spices, if you like. Top with remaining 1 tablespoon grated topping. Enjoy!

Honey Soy Broiled Salmon

Ingredients:

- 1 scallion, minced
- 2 tablespoons reduced-sodium soy sauce
- 1 tablespoon rice vinegar
- 1 tablespoon honey
- 1 teaspoon minced fresh ginger
- 1 pound center-cut salmon fillet, skinned (see Tip) and cut into 4 portions
- 1 teaspoon toasted sesame seeds,

Directions:

1. Whisk scallion, soy sauce, vinegar, honey and ginger in a medium bowl until the honey is dissolved. Place salmon in a sealable plastic bag,
2. Add 3 tablespoons of the sauce and refrigerate; let marinate for 15 minutes. Reserve the remaining sauce.
3. Preheat broiler. Line a small baking pan with foil and coat with cooking spray.
4. Transfer the salmon to the pan, skinned-side down. (Discard the marinade.) Broil the salmon 4 to 6 inches from the heat source until cooked through, 6 to 10

minutes. Drizzle with the reserved sauce and garnish with sesame seeds.

Tips:

How to skin a salmon fillet: Place skin-side down. Starting at the tail end, slip a long knife between the fish flesh and the skin, holding down firmly with your other hand. Gently push the blade along at a 30° angle, separating the fillet from the skin without cutting through either.

To toast sesame seeds, heat a small dry skillet over low heat. Add seeds and stir constantly, until golden and fragrant, about 2 minutes. Transfer to a small bowl and let cool.

People with celiac disease or gluten-sensitivity should use soy sauces that are labeled "gluten-free," as soy sauce may contain wheat or other gluten-containing sweeteners and flavors.

Chicken and Asparagus Stir fry

Serves 4

Ingredients:

- 1 1/2 pounds skinless chicken breast, cut into 1-inch cubes
- Kosher salt, to taste
- 1/2 cup reduced-sodium chicken broth
- 2 tablespoons reduced-sodium shoyu or soy sauce (or Tamari for GF)
- 2 teaspoons cornstarch
- 2 tablespoons water
- 1 tbsp canola or grapeseed oil, divided
- 1 bunch asparagus, ends trimmed, cut into 2-inch pieces
- 6 cloves garlic, chopped
- 1 tbsp fresh ginger
- 3 tablespoons fresh lemon juice
- fresh black pepper, to taste

Directions:

1. Lightly season the chicken with salt. In a small bowl, combine chicken broth and soy sauce. In a second small bowl combine the cornstarch and water and mix well to combine.

2. Heat a large non-stick wok over medium-high heat, when hot add 1 teaspoon of the oil, then add the asparagus and cook until tender-crisp, about 3 to 4 minutes. Add the garlic and ginger and cook until golden, about 1 minute. Set aside.

3. Increase the heat to high, then add 1 teaspoon of oil and half of the chicken and cook until browned and cooked through, about 4 minutes on each side. Remove and set aside and repeat with the remaining oil and chicken. Set aside.

4. Add the soy sauce mixture; bring to a boil and cook about 1-1/2 minutes. Add lemon juice and cornstarch mixture and stir well, when it simmers return the chicken and asparagus to the wok and mix well, remove from heat and serve.

5. Heat a large non-stick wok over medium-high heat, when hot add 1 teaspoon of the oil, then add the asparagus and cook until tender-crisp, about 3 to 4 minutes. Add the garlic and ginger and cook until golden, about 1 minute. Set aside.

6. Increase the heat to high, then add 1 teaspoon of oil and half of the chicken and cook until browned and

cooked through, about 4 minutes on each side. Remove and set aside and repeat with the remaining oil and chicken. Set aside.

7. Add the soy sauce mixture; bring to a boil and cook about 1-1/2 minutes. Add lemon juice and cornstarch mixture and stir well, when it simmers return the chicken and asparagus to the wok and mix well, remove from heat and serve.

Shawarma Chicken Bowls with Basil-Lemon Vinaigrette

Serves 4

Ingredients:

Chicken Shawarma

- 1 lb / 453 gr free-range organic chicken breast, cut into 3-inch strips
- 2 tablespoons olive oil
- 2 tablespoons lemon juice
- ¾ teaspoon fine grain sea salt
- 3 garlic cloves, minced
- 1 teaspoon curry powder
- ½ teaspoon ground cumin
- ¼ teaspoon ground coriander

Salad

- 6 cups / 3.5 oz / 100 gr spring greens
- 1 cup / 5.3 oz / 150 gr cherry tomatoes, halved
- 2 handfuls torn fresh basil leaves
- 1 avocado, sliced

Basil-Lemon Vinaigrette

- 2 large handfuls fresh basil leaves
- 1 clove garlic, smashed
- ½ teaspoon fine grain sea salt
- 2 tablespoons fresh lemon juice
- 5 tablespoons olive oil
- 6 cups / 3.5 oz / 100 gr spring greens
- 1 cup / 5.3 oz / 150 gr cherry tomatoes, halved
- 2 handfuls torn fresh basil leaves
- 1 avocado, sliced

Directions:

1. In a bowl whisk olive oil, lemon juice, garlic, salt, curry powder, cumin and coriander until combined.
2. In a shallow sealable container or in a large Ziploc bag, combine chicken strips and marinade.
3. Cover or seal and marinate in the refrigerator for at least 20 minutes (marinate overnight for fullest flavor.)
4. When you're ready to make the meal, heat a large nonstick skillet over medium-high heat.
5. Add a tiny bit of olive oil, add the chicken and cook until golden brown and cooked through, about 6 to 8 minutes turning regularly, until juices run clear.
6. In the meantime make the vinaigrette. In a food processor (or small blender), process the basil, garlic,

salt, and lemon juice until smooth. With the motor running, slowly add the oil. Blend until combined. Set aside.

7. To make the salads, add the greens in a large bowl and toss them with a sprinkle of salt and pepper. Add the chicken on top along with the tomatoes, basil, and avocado.

8. Drizzle the bowl with the basil-lemon vinaigrette and serve.

Spaghetti Squash Noodle Bowl with Lime Peanut Sauce

Serves 4

Ingredients:

Squash noodle

- 1 large spaghetti squash, cut in half lengthwise + seeds scooped out
- 4 kale stalks, stems removed
- 1 shallot, peeled
- 1/2 cup chopped toasted nuts of your preference (cashews)
- 3 tbsp sesame seeds (toasted, raw)
- chopped leafy herb if you like (cilantro, mint, thai basil etc)
- 1 bunch of broccoli, cut into florets
- salt + pepper

Lime peanut sauce

- 1/2 inch fresh ginger, peeled + rough chopped
- 2 cloves of garlic, peeled + rough chopped
- 1-2 tsp sriracha (or other hot sauce you like)

- 2 tbsp peanut butter (or tahini, sunflower seed butter, almond butter etc)
- 1 lime, peeled + chopped
- 1 tbsp rice vinegar
- 2 tsp agave nectar
- 1 tbsp tamari soy sauce
- little scoop of extra virgin coconut oil (optional)
- 1/4 tsp toasted sesame oil
- 1/2 cup grapeseed oil

Directions:

1. Preheat the oven to 375 degrees F.
2. Line a baking sheet with parchment and place the squash halves, cut side down, onto the sheet. Bake for about an hour or until the flesh pulls away in easy strands.
3. While the squash is baking, slice the kale leaves into 1/3-inch ribbons and place in a large bowl. Cut the shallot in half lengthwise, slice the halves into thin half-moons and set aside. Chop up the herbs and toasted nuts as well, set them aside with the shallows.
4. Once you've cut the broccoli, set a medium saucepan with about an inch of water over medium heat. Bring it to a simmer. Place the broccoli florets into a steamer basket and set aside until right before service.

5. Place all of the sauce ingredients in a blender and blend until fully incorporated. Taste for seasoning and set aside.

6. When squash is cool enough to handle, place the steamer basket of broccoli into the pot with the simmering water. Put a lid on it and allow broccoli to steam for 3-4 minutes, or desired doneness. While broccoli is steaming, scrape the spaghetti strands out with a fork into the large bowl with the sliced kale. The heat from the squash should wilt the kale slightly. Pour a big splash of the dressing into the bowl, season with salt and pepper and lightly toss the squash and kale.

7. Remove broccoli from the heat. Portion the squash and kale into 4 bowls. Top each bowl with the steamed broccoli, sliced shallots, chopped nuts, sesame seeds, chopped herbs and extra sauce.

Dinner Recipes

Cheeseburger Casserole

Serves 6

Ingredients:

Casserole

- 5 slices bacon, chopped
- 2 lbs ground sirloin, lean
- ½ teaspoon chili powder
- ½ teaspoon garlic powder
- ½ teaspoon salt
- ¼ teaspoon pepper
- 1 egg
- 8 ounces Italian cheese blend (or cheddar or your favorite)

Directions:

1. Preheat oven to 350 degrees F .
2. Place the bacon in a frying pan and cook over medium heat for 5-7 minutes.
3. Add ground beef to pan and cook until both are browned.

4. Season with chili powder, garlic powder, salt and pepper.
5. Add the egg and1/2 of the cheese.
6. Press the meat mixture into a greased 2-quart casserole dish.
7. Top with remaining cheese.
8. Bake, uncovered, for 35 minutes, until hot and bubbly.
9. Serve topped with garnishes of your choice.

Garnish

- 2 cups lettuce, shredded
- 1 cup sour cream
- ¼ cup hot sauce

Low Carb Herb-Crusted Lamb Chops

Serves 2

Ingredients:

- 2 large cloves garlic, smashed, or 1½ teaspoons jarred garlic
- 1 sprig fresh thyme, snipped
- 1 sprig fresh rosemary, snipped
- 1 teaspoon kosher salt
- 1 tablespoon extra-virgin olive oil
- 4 1¼ inch lamb loin chops

Directions:

1. Smash the garlic and snip the herbs (leave the stems behind first). Mix them with the salt and half the olive oil in a large bowl. Add the lamb chops, turning them to coat them. Stick the bowl in the fridge and leave them to marinate for half an hour. Or do this a few hours ahead of time to get a jump start on dinner.
2. About 25 minutes before you want to serve them, preheat oven to 400° F. Put the rest of the olive oil into a saucepan with an oven-proof handle and heat

on high. Add the chops and brown them on both sides, about 3 minutes per side.

3. Then place pan in the oven and roast the lamb chops until they're the way you like them. Medium rare is about 10 minutes. When done, transfer them to serving plates and let them rest 5 minutes before serving

Roasted Barramundi with Tomato and Olive Relish

Serves 2

Ingredients:

- 2 fillets Barramundi (or other mild white fish), about 5-6 oz. each
- 2 tsp. olive oil, for rubbing fish
- 2 tsp. Szeged Fish Rub, for rubbing fish
- 1/4 cup finely chopped cherry tomatoes
- 1/4 cup finely chopped black olives
- 1/4 cup finely chopped green olives
- 1 T lemon zest
- 2 T fresh-squeezed lemon juice (zest the lemon first, and then squeeze the juice)
- 2 T finely chopped fresh parsley
- 1 T olive oil
- salt and fresh ground black pepper to taste

Directions:
1. Let fish thaw overnight or all day in the refrigerator. If your fillets have a flap of very thin fish on the side,

trim that off because it will get overcooked by the time the thicker parts are done.

2. Turn on the oven or toaster oven to 400F/200C. Rub both sides of the fish with olive oil and sprinkle with Szeged Fish Rub, rubbing it into the fish, and put fish on a roasting sheet. Let the fish come to room temperature while the oven heats and while you prepare the relish.

3. Finely chop the cherry tomatoes, black olives, and green olives. Zest the lemon and then squeeze the juice and measure out 2 tablespoons lemon juice. (Just freeze the extra lemon juice if you have some.) Chops 2 tablespoons of flat or curly parsley. Stir together the tomatoes, black olives, green olives, lemon zest, lemon juice and olive oil and season the relish with a tiny amount of salt and fresh-ground black pepper.

4. When the fish is room temperature, put it into the oven or toaster oven and roast 10-12 minutes, or just until it's barely firm to the touch. Serve hot, with a generous serving of the tomato and olive relish spooned over.

Low Carb Italian Shrimp

Serves 1

Ingredients:

- 1 garlic clove, chopped
- 2 tablespoons olive oil
- ½ teaspoon salt
- ½ teaspoon oregano
- 1 pound Daily Chef™ Cooked Medium Shrimp
- ¼ cup Olive Garden Signature Italian Dressing

Directions:
1. Follow defrosting instructions on bag.
2. Heat sauté pan on medium heat. Add olive oil to pan.
3. Add garlic and shrimp. Make sure shrimp is on an even layer in the pan.
4. Stir shrimp and re-arrange them, making sure to cook both sides. Remove mixture from pan once tender and lightly crisped, about 2-5 minutes.
5. Toss shrimp with Olive Garden dressing and seasonings. Serve with desired sides.

Oven-Fried Chicken

Ingredients:

- 1/3 cup low-fat buttermilk
- 1/4 cup finely chopped fresh chives
- 1 teaspoon Dijon mustard
- 1/4 teaspoon hot sauce
- 4 bone-in chicken breasts
- 1/2 cup dried breadcrumbs
- 1/2 teaspoon salt
- 1/2 teaspoon freshly ground pepper

Directions:
1. In a medium bowl, whisk together the buttermilk, chives, mustard, and hot sauce. Remove the skin from the chicken breasts, add the chicken to the bowl, and let it soak for at least 30 minutes or overnight.
2. Preheat the oven to 425°F. Spray a rimmed baking sheet with cooking spray. Place the breadcrumbs in a wide, shallow bowl.
3. Remove the chicken from the marinade, and season it with salt and pepper.
4. Dip the chicken into the breadcrumbs, and toss well to coat. Place the chicken on the prepared baking sheet.

5. Spray the chicken generously with cooking spray, and bake until it is just cooked through, 25 to 30 minutes.

Snacks Recipes

Skillet Pizza

Serves 1

Ingredients:

- Handful of shredded mozzarella cheese - just enough to cover the bottom of a 10-inch skillet
- 1-2 tablespoons canned crushed tomatoes (no sugar added)
- Pepperoni slices
- Garlic powder
- Italian seasoning or dried basil
- Crushed red pepper, Parmesan cheese, and fresh basil (optional)

Directions:
1. Heat small, nonstick skillet over medium.
2. Cover the bottom of hot skillet evenly with shredded mozzarella cheese.
3. Lightly spread the crushed tomatoes on top of the cheese, using the back of a spoon, and leaving a border around the edges of the cheese crust.

4. Sprinkle with garlic powder and dried basil or Italian seasoning. Arrange pepperoni on top.

5. Cook until sizzling, bubbled, and edges are brown. Try to lift up the edges of the pizza with a spatula. When it is ready, it will easily lift up from the pan. If it sticks, that means it's not quite ready. Keep lifting and checking frequently. When it finally starts to lift up easily without sticking, work spatula gently and slowly underneath to loosen up entire pizza and transfer to a cutting board.

6. Sprinkle lightly with Parmesan, fresh torn basil leaves, and crushed red pepper, if desired.

7. Allow to cool for about 5 minutes. The crust will firm up even more while it cools. Cut with a pizza cutter, transfer to a serving plate, and enjoy!

Pepperoni Chips

Ingredients:

- 1 package of (regular or turkey) pepperonis

Directions:

1. Layer two paper towels and place as many pepperonis on top of it as desired, making sure they don't overlap. Cover with an additional paper towel.

2. Microwave the pepperonis until they are stiff and crispy, usually no more than 1 minute.

3. Repeat the entire process for additional pepperoni chips. Serve with low carb dip or even my favorite, salsa!

Pizza Zucchinis

Ingredients:

- 1 zucchini, washed well and ends cut off
- ¼ cup spaghetti sauce
- 1 cup shredded mozzarella

Directions:

1. Preheat oven to 350 degrees.
2. Spray cooking spray (or lightly wipe olive oil on baking sheet).
3. Slice zucchini into ¼" slices and place on baking sheet.
4. Spread sauce on top of slices.
5. Top with mozzarella cheese and any other pizza topping you'd like.
6. Bake until cheese is melted and golden brown, remove and cool.
7. Enjoy!

Zero Carb Cheesy Egg Chips

Serves 1

Ingredients:

- 4 Egg Whites
- 2 tbsp shredded cheese of your flavor choice
- 1/2 tbsp water to thin it out a little
- Salt and pepper to taste if desired

Directions:

1. Preheat your oven to 400 degrees and get ready a non-stick medium size muffin pan
2. Whisk together your egg whites, water, and whatever seasoning you want to flavor
3. With a syringe, fill each muffin cup with approx 2.5ml of the egg white mixture, needs to be just enough to cover the bottom.
4. Sprinkle a small pinch of the cheese you desire onto each egg white
5. Bake for 15 minutes to acquire a good crunch without burning, but check them every couple of minutes to make sure.

6. Remove from oven once they are at your preferred crunch, and enjoy them with any low carb dip or solely on their own.

Cheesy Cauliflower Breadsticks

Serves 8

Ingredients:

- •4 cups of riced cauliflower (about 1 large head of cauliflower)
- •4 eggs
- •2 cups of mozzarella cheese
- •3 tsp oregano
- •4 cloves garlic, minced
- •salt and pepper to taste
- •1 to 2 cups mozzarella cheese (for topping)

Directions:

1. Preheat oven to 425 F degrees. Prepare 2 pizza dishes or a large baking sheet with parchment paper.
2. Make sure your cauliflower is roughly chopped in florets. Add the florets to your food processor and pulse until cauliflower resembles rice.
3. Place the cauliflower in a microwavable container and cover with lid. Microwave for 10 minutes. Place the microwaved cauliflower in a large bowl and add the 4

eggs, 2 cups of mozzarella, oregano, garlic and salt and pepper. Mix everything together.

4. Separate the mixture in half and place each half onto the prepared baking sheets and shape into either a pizza crust, or a rectangular shape for the breadsticks.

5. Bake the crust (no topping yet) for about 25 minutes or until nice and golden. Don't be afraid the crust is not soggy at all. Once golden, sprinkle with remaining mozzarella cheese and put back in the oven for another 5 minutes or until cheese has melted.

6. Slice and serve.

Conclusion

I hope that through this book you have learned how to practice the low carb and high protein diet on your own. Keep in mind your checklist of low carb or high protein content food items; you can bring this list on your next trip to the grocery. With your knowledge on computing your BMI and comparing it with the ideal ranges, you can target your desired body weight.

I hope you can also try the recommended recipes listed on this book to jumpstart your low carb diet lifestyle. Take note, these are just few of the many recipes out there and the recipes that you can develop yourself. Be creative with the low carb and high protein food groups, this way you can still taste the flavors you want while shedding the weight that you dislike.

The next step after reading this book is for you to go to your pantry or kitchen. Begin to stock up on your low carb and high protein food ingredients that you can use for your recipes. At the same time, remove non-low carb diet friendly ingredients, this way you can remove the temptation from using them. Consider bringing in home cooked meals to your place of work. Most of the food being served in your cafeteria may not pass the low carb requirements of your diet.

A few days before you start the diet, begin to ease out of your usual carb loading. Choose lean meat food when you order, or avoid high carb content snacks in the office. This way when you begin the full diet on Day 1, you are more than ready. This will avoid crashes, which are common to those who start a diet unprepared.

With the low carb and high protein diet, your dream of achieving your desired weight can truly become a reality! Start practicing the low carb diet lifestyle and start cooking the low carb recipes today!

SARAH E. DAWSON

Final Thoughts...

Thank you again for buying this book!

Finally, if you received value from this book, please take the time to share your thoughts and post a review on Amazon.com. It'd be greatly appreciated!

Thank you and good luck!

Check Out My Other Books

Below you'll find some of my best-selling books that are popular on Amazon and Kindle as well. Simply go to the URL below to check them out.

http://bit.ly/sarahdawson

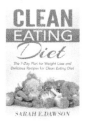 Clean Eating Diet: The 7-Day Plan for Weight Loss and Delicious Recipes for Clean Eating Diet

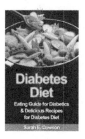 Diabetes Diet: Eating Guide for Diabetics and Delicious Recipes for Diabetes Diet

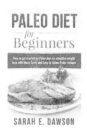 Paleo Diet For Beginners: How to Get Started on Paleo Diet for Effective Weight Loss with these Tasty and Easy-to-follow Paleo Recipes

Made in the USA
Coppell, TX
14 April 2023